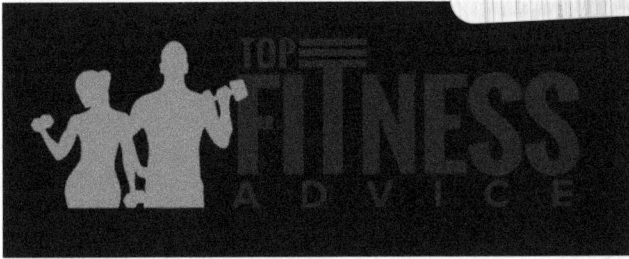

TOP FITNESS ADVICE

HEALTH

How These 50 Everyday Changes Can Boost Your Health, Increase Your Energy & Make You Live Longer!

Kayla Bates

ink

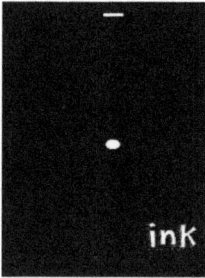

For more information about the contents of this book or questions to the author, please contact Kayla Bates at kayla@topfitnessadvice.com

Disclaimer

This book provides wellness management information in an informative and educational manner only, with information that is general in nature and that is not specific to you, the reader. The contents of this book are intended to assist you and other readers in your personal wellness efforts. Consult your physician regarding the applicability of any information provided in this book to you.

Nothing in this book should be construed as personal advice or diagnosis, and must not be used in this manner. The information provided about conditions is general in nature. This information does not cover all possible uses, actions, precautions, side-effects, or interactions of medicines, or medical procedures. The information in this book should not be considered as complete and does not cover all diseases, ailments, physical conditions, or their treatment.

You should consult with your physician before beginning any exercise, weight loss, or health care program. This book should not be used in place of a call or visit to a competent health-care professional. You should consult a health care professional before adopting any of the suggestions in this book or before drawing inferences from it.

Any decision regarding treatment and medication for your condition should be made with the advice and consultation of a qualified health care professional. If you have, or suspect you have, a health-care problem, then you should immediately contact a qualified health care professional for treatment.

No Warranties: The author and publisher don't guarantee or warrant the quality, accuracy, completeness, timeliness, appropriateness or suitability of the information in this book, or of any product or services referenced in this book.

The information in this book is provided on an "as is" basis and the author and publisher make no representations or warranties of any kind with respect to this information. This book may contain inaccuracies, typographical errors, or other errors.

Table of Contents

Would you prefer to listen to my book, rather than read it?

Download the audiobook version for free!

If you go to the special link below and sign up to Audible as a new customer, you can get the audiobook version of my book completely free.

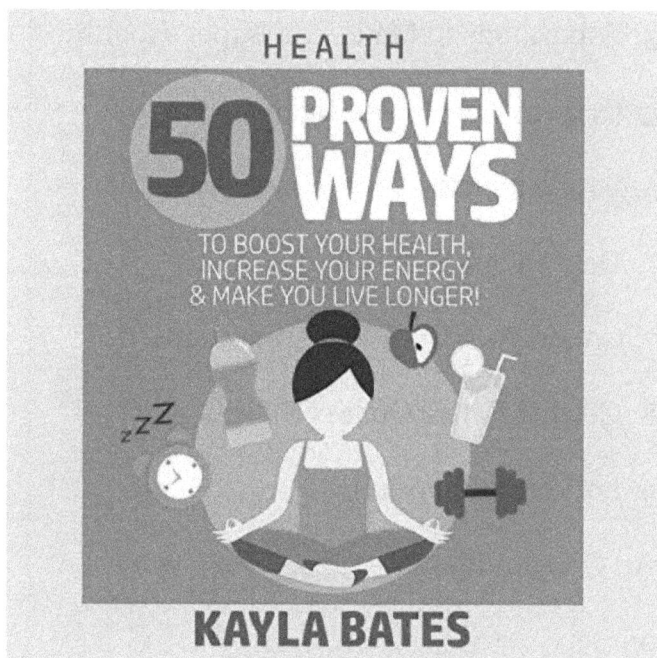

Go here to get your audiobook version for free:

TopFitnessAdvice.com/go/Health50

Who is the Book For?

This book is for anyone who feels like they are not living their fullest, healthiest life. For the person who though not physically ill, cannot be classified as well either.

If you cannot remember the last time that you woke up fully refreshed after a good night's sleep. If you find that you have fewer reserves of energy to fall back on. Or if you simply feel that there has got to be a better way to live your life, this book is for you.

Anyone will benefit from the changes that this book advises. But those who will benefit most will be those who have let their healthy habits slide a little. Whether for convenience or because we didn't know better, we all have slips once in a while.

This book will help you to turn this situation around so that those slips don't do permanent damage.

What Will This Book Teach You?

There is a lot of information in this book. When it comes to absolute health and vitality, it is not simply enough to eat the right foods and exercise. This will help but you need to take a more holistic view – you need to look at changing your mindset and improving your overall quality of life as well.

This book aims to help you do that. You will learn how to get back that glowing health and vitality you had in your youth.

You will learn what supplements should be taken daily. What superfoods you should eat. What the worst possible food to eat is. Using herbal teas as natural remedies and about how to keep properly hydrated. You will learn how to spice up your life and some ancient secrets to wellness.

You will learn how to get the best bang for your buck when it comes to exercise. You will learn simple exercises that are highly effective. Exercises that will help you trim and tone yourself and naturally improve your energy levels.

You will learn how to change your mindset so that you become calmer, more focused and generally more content. Daily exercises will help you feel more content without needing to win the lottery.

You will learn how to clear your body of the myriad of toxins that assail it on a daily basis. Toxins that leach energy and vitality and contribute to premature aging.

We will also go through improving the quality of your sleep – one of the most important overall health and beauty treatments that we can access.

We have devoted a section on how you can create your own personal spa treatments. We all deserve to be spoilt at times but it is not always possible to book into a spa. Recreate the benefits in your own home.

Learn skin care tricks for a natural radiance – learn how to care for the skin from the outside and the inside.

Introduction

Are you tired most of the time? Have you lost the pep in your step? Modern day living takes its toll – eating on the go, ditching the gym and working too hard is very hard on your body.

Years of this kind of abuse have resulted in many of us literally being the walking wounded. Why we are not actually physically ill, we are also not as vital as we should be.

Do you want to start reclaiming your vitality? Do want better health and more energy?

The good news is that it is never too late to start. You can make a big difference to your health in a very short time. And it really isn't that hard.

In this book, we will go through fifty steps that you can take in order to recover your health and vitality. Each step, done on its own, will contribute to making you feel better in a hurry. The cumulative effect of all the steps together is going to change your life completely.

Read through the whole book once first and then start with the tips that you feel will be easiest for you.

I realize that you want to get started straight away and work through the steps as fast as possible but I urge you to reconsider. Incorporate only one from each chapter to start off with and work your way up from there.

The reason for taking it a bit more slowly is that it then becomes a lot easier to incorporate and maintain over the long haul. Once you start to see the positive changes in your life, you will be even more inclined to carry on making changes.

The tips are divided up into ten different sections – what to drink; exercise; superfoods; mental acuity, supplements; detoxing; spa treatments; sleep; lotions and potions and general pick-me-ups.

Each tip has been tried and tested and will help to get you feeling better, looking better, being healthier and living a better quality of life.

Are You ALWAYS Hungry When You Try to Lose Weight?

Discover How to STOP Starving Yourself & Lose Weight FASTER By Eating MORE Food!

For this month only, you can get Kayla's best-selling & most popular book absolutely free – *The Ultimate Guide to Healthy Eating & Losing Weight Without Starving Yourself!*

Get Your FREE Copy Here:

TopFitnessAdvice.com/Book

Discover how you can **start eating MORE food** and see weight loss results faster than ever before. Learn about the 10 most powerful fat-burning foods and how they boost the rate that your body burns fat. And last but not least, finally put an end to your emotional or "bored" eating habits. With this book, readers were able to significantly improve their weight loss results. So, it's highly recommended that you get this book, especially while it's free!

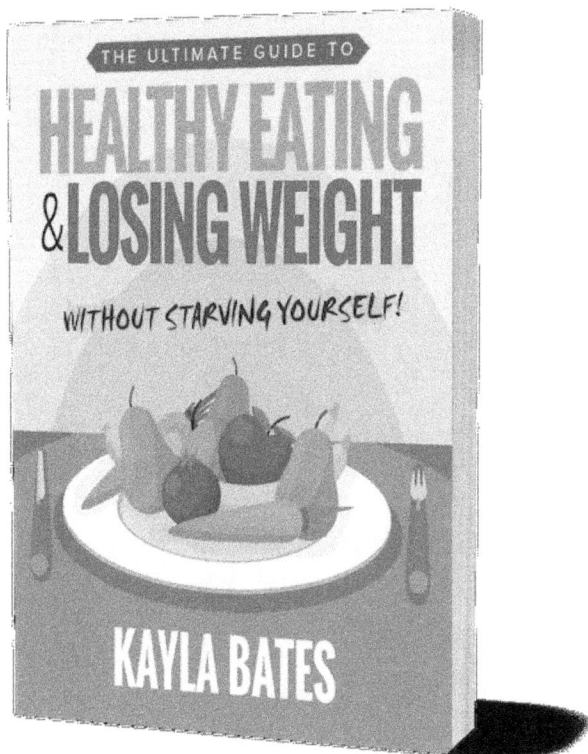

Get Your FREE Copy Here:

TopFitnessAdvice.com/Book

Chapter 1

Drink Your Way to Better Health

We all know that water is one of the essentials when it comes to good health. And yes, one of the tips here is going to be to drink more water. But there is so much more that you can do to become completely healthy. You can make smoothies, juice veggies, make your own flavored water, etc.

You can tailor your daily water intake in such a way that you get the maximum amount of goodness with it. And in this chapter, I'll show you how to do that.

Tip 1: Drink the Right Amount of Water for Your Weight

Conventional wisdom holds that we should drink between six and eight glasses of water a day. Research has shown that even this may not be enough.

In order to determine how much water you should drink, a simple calculation is in order:

(Your weight in pounds) x 2/3 = Base amount of water to drink a day in ounces. Finally, add another 12 ounces of water for every half an hour of exercise that you do. So, if you weigh 130 pounds, for example, and did a half an hour of exercise a day, the calculation would look like this:

130 x 2/3 = 86 ounces of water.

Add in the 12 ounces for the half an hour of exercise and you get a total of 98.

There are 8 ounces in a glass so that means that your intake should be twelve and a quarter glasses of water. See how the six to eight glasses recommended falls short?

The easiest way to increase your water intake is to keep a bottle or jug of water near you at all times. Force yourself to drink a glass of water every hour, if that is what it takes.

Tip 2: Start the Day Alkalizing Your Body

Our modern diets contain a lot of foods that cause acidity in the body. Red meat, trans-fats, and refined carbs, to name but a few, can all upset the pH balance of your body.

Now, if this happened just once in a while, it would not be such a big issue. If this continues, however, the higher levels of acidity in the body start doing damage.

You see, the body does need some acidity but when there is too much, the body has to work that much harder to rid itself of the excess. This, in addition to the stress that most of us are already under leads to a build-up of inflammation in the body.

Now again, the inflammatory response is something that the body needs. It is what the body uses to heal itself. It is, however, meant to be a short-term measure.

If the inflammatory response is activated continuously over a long period of time, it becomes extremely harmful to the body. This leads to disease and fatigue.

Think of it for a minute – the inflammatory response is like your own personal army and very effective if brought to bear occasionally. Now, let's say that you make the soldiers fight every day – they will quickly become fatigued and a lot less effective.

One thing that you can do starting now to help your body is to start your day by alkalizing it.

For now, I just want you to do one thing. When you get up in the morning, before you do anything else, take a glass of warm water and add the juice of half a lemon or two tablespoons of apple cider vinegar. Drink while still warm.

Tip 3: Have a Smoothie to Start Your Day

I don't know about you, but I do battle when it comes to eating the right amount of vegetables and fruit. Personally, I prefer a cheeseburger and chips to a plateful of veggies any day.

And that is why I have a smoothie for breakfast every morning. Not only do they taste great, but they are packed with nutrients. And, when made right, they will help to keep you going all the way through to lunchtime.

The basic recipe that I use for a smoothie is simple:

- ½ cup of milk of your choice (I like almond milk)

- ½ cup of yoghurt or a scoop of protein powder
- 1 banana (Adds a nice creamy texture and sweetens the smoothie)
- 1 other serving of fruit – if it is a hot day, I like to add frozen berries.
- 1 carrot or vegetable of your choice (as long as it can be eaten raw)
- ½ cup of oats
- ½ cup of oat bran
- Water to thin it down if required
- 1 serving of nuts of your choice
- 1 serving of mixed seeds of your choice (like sunflower, pumpkin or linseeds, for example)

Blend everything together until smooth. This does make enough for two servings so I do share with my family. Otherwise, if I know I am going to have a busy day, I store the leftovers in the refrigerator and have another smoothie for lunch.

Tip 4: Freshly Extracted Vegetable Juices

Now I am going to preface this by saying that I feel it is better to have your vegetables in a smoothie because then you get the benefit of the fiber in them as well.

Juicing I reserve for those times when I really need an extra jolt of energy or if I feel as though I am getting sick.

Also, please not that I said vegetable juices here. You can, if you like, add in a low-GI fruit such as an apple to make the drink more palatable but stick to low-GI fruits only.

I also suggest that you drink your juice only with a meal. The reason is simple. With the fiber removed, the juices become a lot easier for your body to convert to glucose. They can, thus, have a significant impact on your blood sugar if you are not careful.

Tip 5: Drink Some Tea

Coffee does have its uses but you can get a lot more benefits by drinking tea. In this instance, I am referring to green tea and herbal teas. These teas are not only healthier for you, they give you a boost without making you feel all jittery.

I have an extensive herb garden and so I have my pick of fresh herbs to pick for my tea. If you don't have a garden, try to grow herbs on the windowsill so that you always have a fresh supply.

Here are my favorite teas and ones that you should consider:

- **Green Tea**: Green tea is packed with anti-oxidants and will give you a very nice boost of energy. The tea, if consumed on a regular basis will not only nourish you but also help you to lose weight.

- **Rooibos/ Red Bush Tea**: This tea contains no caffeine at all and is perfectly safe for babies to drink. It calms and soothes the mind and packs a punch when it comes to anti-oxidant content.

- **Mint Tea**: This is one of my go-to teas when I need a quick pick-me-up; when I have indigestion or heartburn and when I feel a touch of a cold/ flu coming on. (And it tastes great.) It is also good for detoxing.

There are many other herbal teas that you can choose from. Do yourself a favor and do some research into what you do and don't like.

Chapter 2

Put More Pep in Your Step with Exercise

I can almost hear the groans with this one. Exercise is not always a favorite pastime – I know that I hated going to the gym. I also got sick of everyone to nag me to do more exercise.

The reason that this particular piece of advice keeps coming up is simple, it works.

Your body was made to move, believe it or not, your rump wasn't designed to sit on all day.

Fortunately getting more exercise can be done quite easily.

Tip 6: Do a Sun Salutation in the Morning

This is best done before breakfast and is a yoga move that will work every muscle in your body. The exercise is simple and requires very little in the way of physical fitness.

The picture below shows the sequence that should be followed. Don't worry if you cannot quite stretch as far as she does – you will improve over time.

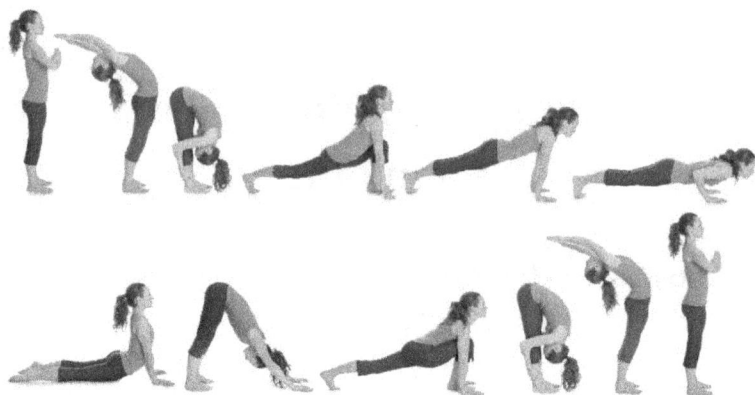

Tip 7: Rebound Your Way to Health

Get yourself a mini-trampoline and start bouncing on it every day. I like the mini-trampoline because it is a lot more fun than going to the gym.

Don't be fooled, though, you do get a great workout at the same time. When I started, I could barely manage to do two or three minutes.

The mini-trampoline allows you to get a cardiovascular workout. You can also use it as a substitute for a treadmill at a push. You can march or run in place on the mini-trampoline if you like. Walking or running this way is more of a workout and does not place nearly as much stress on your joints.

I recommend working up to two fifteen minute sessions a day – one before breakfast and one when you get home after work.

Just don't rebound too close to bedtime or you might find that it is harder to sleep.

Tip 8: Sneak Exercise In

How many times have you said something along the lines of, "I don't have time to exercise." This is never entirely true.

I know – I used the same excuse myself. And, if you look at it from the point of needing to get dressed, go to the gym, shower, etc. it does take up a fair amount of time.

You do not have to spend an hour a day in the gym to feel the benefits of exercise. The basic recommended exercise levels to stay healthy are half an hour of exercise that raises the heartbeat at least five times a week. You don't even have to get it all in one go.

If you look at it this way, you have plenty of time to exercise and it is easy to sneak it in.

Start by seeing how you can work exercise into your daily routine.

When you are brushing your teeth, for example, use the time to do squats or lunges.

When you are sitting at your desk, do some foot rolls or butt crunches.

Choose a trigger point, like being at a red stoplight, and pull your stomach in every time you pass that trigger point.

Jog to your mailbox instead of walking.

Tip 9: Find Exercise that Feels Like Play

Maybe you don't like to do aerobics. Maybe you don't like running. That's fine. Avoid them completely. But do find some form of exercise that you enjoy doing. Take dancing, for example, it is a lot more fun than sitting on the rowing machine and can be just as effective.

If you want to make exercise an integral part of your day, you need to start looking for ways to make it feel like play. The more fun you have, the more likely you are to stick with it.

Think back to when you were a child – were there any sports that you enjoyed playing? What did you love to play at as a child? Take your cue from this and see where that takes you.

Do try different things until you find something that you like. Make being able to exercise as effortless as possible for you and it will soon be something that you look forward to doing.

Look for something that you could do at home, if you like.

Tip 10: Get an Exercise Buddy

Having someone to exercise with can make a lot of difference, especially if you are worried that you might slack off.

It's one thing to slack off on your own but quite another when you slack off if you are accountable to someone else.

Exercising with a buddy is useful because you can motivate each other. It can also make the time go by faster if you have someone that you can exercise with.

When choosing your exercise buddy, be sure to choose someone who will be as committed to the program as you are. It will also be better if they are of a similar fitness level to you.

I hope that you are enjoying this book so far, and if you could spare 30 seconds, I would greatly appreciate you leaving a review on Amazon.com.

Chapter 3

Superfoods to Make You Super-Healthy

Rev up the nutrient content of your diet by adding in some of the following superfoods. Please note, these are superfoods that might look ordinary at first glance but that pack a powerful punch.

Tip 11: Coconut

Coconut oil has been receiving a lot of press lately. It is a healthy oil that is very stable at high temperature. What this means is that it does not oxidize as easily as other oils and so is not prone to developing free radicals when heated.

Coconut oil is good for cooking with. Fresh coconut or unsweetened coconut flakes are great for your overall health.

Fresh coconut makes for a wonderful snack – it has a high fat content but considering that this is a very healthy fat, that is alright. The fats in coconut will help you shift the extra weight that you have been carrying.

In fact, studies conducted on the benefits of coconut oil found that it could promote weight loss. The participants in the study changed nothing in their diet but added two tablespoons of coconut oil a day.

You can easily do the same by cooking with it or eating the fresh fruit.

Have coconut with some nuts or yogurt and you have a snack that will not only help you lose weight but give you a store of energy as well.

Alternatively, you can use dried coconut, as long as it has not been sweetened.

Tip 12: Blueberries

Blueberries are full of phytoflavinoids and antioxidants, in addition to Vitamin C and potassium. This makes them one of the best tools against inflammation and ill-health that you can get.

They can, in addition to the anti-inflammatory benefits, also reduce your chances of developing cancer and heart disease. All you need is about half a cup a day to start seeing benefits.

Eat them as they are if you like or stir into your morning bowl of oats. A breakfast of oats (the non-instant kind), yogurt and blueberries will keep you going until it is time for lunch.

You can have the odd blueberry muffin but don't rely on that to get your daily dose.

First of all, a muffin or two will not have a sufficient quantity of blueberries. Second of all, the ingredients that go into the muffin make it a less than healthy treat.

Tip 13: Oily Fish

The Omega-3 content in the fish will help to reduce inflammation, keep your skin and joints healthy, help you maintain your memory and protect your heart.

We don't actually need a lot of Omega-3's in our diet. The problem is that most of us eat too much in terms of Omega-6's.

Now whilst Omega-6's also have a place in our diets, it can cause inflammation when consumed in doses that are too high.

Research suggests that we should eat about the same quantity of Omega-3's and Omega-6's. The average American, however, eats about sixteen times more Omega-6s than Omega-3's. It's a disaster waiting to happen.

Getting enough Omega-3's in the diet can be surprisingly difficult if you do not eat enough oily fish like salmon, mackerel or sardines. All you need is to replace two or three meals containing red meat with those containing oily fish to see the benefits.

Walnuts and flaxseeds also have high levels of Omega-3's in them but our bodies are not as easily able to convert plant sources of this nutrient to a useable form. As a result, you are better off eating the fish.

Tip 14: Fiber

Again, this is probably a tip that you have heard before. What I will bet you weren't aware of, however, is exactly how important fiber is. Fiber comes in two forms – soluble and insoluble. The body cannot digest either form of fiber so they pass through into the intestine undigested.

Why have fiber at all then? Fiber plays a vital role when it comes to balancing your blood sugar levels. It slows down the rate at which the body is able to convert your food into glucose. This enables you to have a steadier flow of energy rather than frequent energy spikes.

In addition, fiber helps to mop up excess bad cholesterol, helps you feel fuller for longer and feeds the beneficial microbes in the gut. All of which is important to help you maintain your health.

Adding more fiber to your diet is quite easily accomplished. If you are not accustomed to eating fiber, start adding it back in slowly to minimize discomfort while your body is adjusting.

We should be eating around about 25g of fiber a day, or about 14g of fiber for every 1000 calories that makes up our diet.

If you have tried the smoothie recipe, you are already on the way there. To up fiber intake, swap out refined foods for whole ones where possible.

Tip 15: Oats

Oats are one of mother nature's best superfoods. Whilst the instant varieties do not have nearly the same nutrient power of the less-refined varieties, they can still be healthy.

If you really want to score points, though, look for steel cut oats. They take longer to prepare than instant but they have more fiber, protein, and nutrients.

Alternatively, get yourself some oat bran and add it to the instant oats to rev up the health factor.

Oats are low GI, high in fiber and contain a good quantity of protein – making them perfect as a breakfast food.

For a quick breakfast, soak a cup of oats overnight in a ¾ cup of milk/ water and a ¾ cup of yogurt.

The next morning, stir some of your favorite fruit and some coconut flakes into it and enjoy.

Chapter 4

Getting Your Mind Right

Tip 16: Calming Your Mind

Your mind has so many thoughts whizzing through it all the time and it can be very hard to get it to switch gears and quieten down.

Having some quiet time where you get to completely zone out though is extremely good for you. And the best way to calm your mind is to meditate.

Meditation is a discipline that requires a fair amount of practice but, once you get the hang of it, you'll never do without it again.

There are many ways to meditate and so I encourage you to do some research and find one that suits you. You can gain benefits from meditating for just five minutes a day.

The first time is probably not going to be easy for you. Your mind will want to keep pestering you with thoughts.

The following exercise is extremely useful for beginners because you have something other than your thoughts to concentrate on:

1. Start by sitting comfortably. (Don't lie down or you may fall asleep.) Make sure you will be undisturbed for the next 5-10 minutes.

2. Close your eyes and breathe in deeply to the slow count of five.

3. Hold your breath to the slow count of five.

4. Release your breath to the slow count of five.

5. Repeat as many times as you like – if you find that thoughts are intruding bring your attention back to your breathing again.

6. When you are done, open your eyes and just sit there for a minute or so before moving on with your day.

Tip 17: Spend Time on Gratitude Exercises

If you take only one tip out this book to heart, this should be the one. We, as a society, are very goal orientated. We are taught that we must always strive for success.

Now, there is nothing wrong with striving for success but keeping your eye on the future all the time makes you miss out on what is going on in the present.
We don't take the time to appreciate what we already have because we feel that we should be striving for more.

This attitude can be quite dangerous because we focus on what we are lacking rather than what we have achieved. As a result, there is never a feeling of true contentment in our lives.

If you want to turn things around for you, start by being more grateful for what you do have. Spend a few minutes when you get up in the morning to list five to ten things that you are grateful for.

Last thing at night, go through what you were most grateful for during that day. That way you start and end each day feeling more content.

Tip 18: Change the Way You Treat Others

Now, I am actually referring to how you speak to others. Try to rephrase everything you say so that it has a positive bent to it.

For example, instead of saying, "I am sorry that I am late", you can say, "Thank you for waiting for me." Both examples are correct but the second is more powerful because it has a more positive spin on it.

Try it the next time you go to a store – instead of complaining about how busy the store is, try complimenting the cashier on how well they are dealing with the queue. You will be amazed at the response.

Treat everyone with respect and compassion and, before long, you will find that the world is a much nicer place than you initially though it was.

Tip 19: Start Learning to Use Positive Self-Talk

It is ironic that in life we are usually a good deal harder on ourselves than we ever are on anyone else. How many times have you called yourself an idiot? How many times have you berated yourself for a silly mistake that anyone could have made?

Starting today, cut yourself a bit of slack. Okay, so maybe you'll make mistakes again, but what kind of real damage will that do in the grand scheme of things?

Most of the mistakes that we spend so much time agonizing over have very little impact on our lives in general. Most of the time, they are forgotten about in a few months' time anyway.

Sit down right now and write out what your best qualities are. If you like, ask trusted friends and family members to write what they feel your best qualities are.

Oftentimes what we see as our greatest failings are viewed in a much more positive light by those around us.

Tip 20: Give Yourself Some Easy Wins

Every day we face challenges. Some days are easier than others. Giving yourself some easy wins will help you a great deal when it comes to those really bad days.

Every morning, set yourself a goal or two for that day. Make sure that one of those goals is something that is easily accomplished.

By doing this, you get to experience at least one victory a day, no matter how bad the day is going. It will help to boost your confidence and help you to feel much better about yourself.

Once again, thank you for reading this book, and I hope you're getting a lot of valuable information. I would greatly appreciate it if you could take 30 seconds to leave me a review for this book on Amazon.com.

Enjoying this book?

Check out my other best sellers!

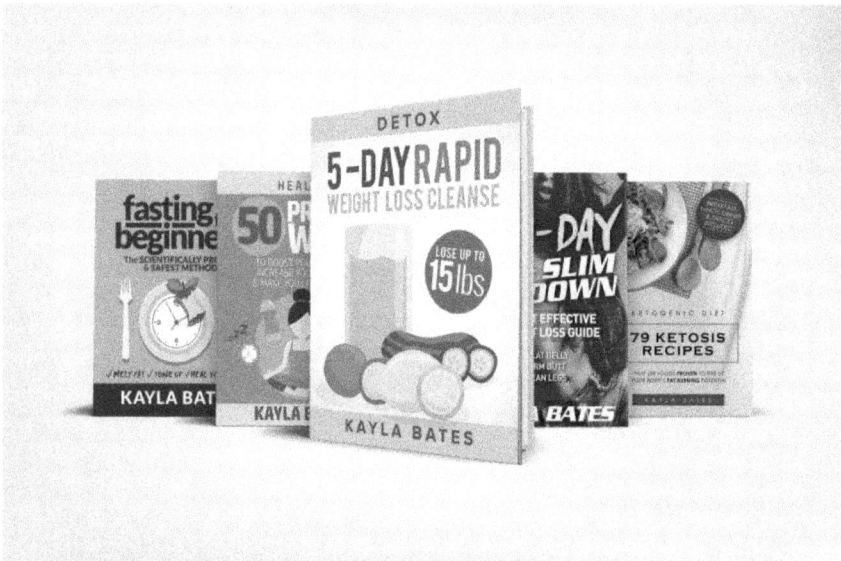

Chapter 5

Supplements - Your Way to Vitality

There are hundreds of supplements on the market today. Trying to keep up with which supplements you should and should not be taking is hard.

Don't waste your money – these are the top five supplements that you should consider.

Tip 21: A Good Quality Multi-Vitamin and Mineral Supplement

Getting all the nutrients that you need from the food that you eat is difficult. A good quality supplement will help to redress some of the deficiencies that you might develop.

That said, it is not a substitute for following a healthy diet. The supplement will not be able to do much good if you keep eating refined foods and sugar that increase the inflammatory response in the body.

Tip 22: Vitamin Sunshine

Vitamin D is one vitamin that a lot of us are deficient in. It's crazy because it is so easy to get the right amount of Vitamin D, even without supplementation.
A long-term deficiency of Vitamin D can make you more prone to depression, developing heart disease, cancer, and diabetes.

Get your daily dose of Vitamin D by standing in full sunlight once a day for about 15 minutes. The more skin you expose, the better. Not such a difficult one, is it?

So why are so many people deficient in this vitamin? Simply because we don't tend to spend a lot of time outdoors during the week anymore. In addition, when we do expose ourselves to the sun, we often make sure that we were sunscreen.

Tip 23: Magnesium

It is no secret that magnesium deficiency is rife. Most people don't even realize that they have a deficiency at all.

Magnesium is one of the minerals that the body needs to produce energy. It is most commonly found in fruits and vegetables and so most of us do not get enough of it in our diets.

In addition, it is essential in order to rid the body of toxins. Insufficient levels of magnesium can lead to irritability, muscle cramps, a higher risk of developing lifestyle disease and a general fatigue.

It is not simply a matter of eating more of the right foods. A lot of fresh produce that is grown nowadays come from magnesium-deficient soil.

Your general state of health can also affect how well the magnesium is absorbed. High levels of highly refined foods and soda can also reduce the amount of magnesium in the body.

If you battle to sleep, take your magnesium supplement just before bed. It has a relaxing and calming effect.

Tip 24: Omega-3's

If you are not someone who likes to eat fish, or you simply do not eat oily fish that often, it is important to supplement your Omega-3 intake.

Choose a salmon oil or cod liver oil supplement for the best results. As mentioned before, vegetarian sources of Omega-3 are not processed very well by the body.

Omega-3's are not called essential fatty acids for nothing. They contribute to the health of your skin, your heart, and help to reduce inflammation throughout your body.

Tip 25: Take Probiotics

Your body has several different strains of bacteria in it. Before you freak out, know that we do need some bacteria to remain healthy.

The good bacteria that are found in your intestines have a significant impact on your wellbeing overall.

They help you to digest your food, they help to boost your immunity and they help to neutralize bacteria that is not good for you. They also prevent you from getting diarrhea.

Recent studies have also shown that those with insufficient numbers of the beneficial bacteria have a higher chance of developing depression.

If you do not have sufficient numbers of the healthy bacteria, the unhealthy bacteria are not kept in check. This can result in poor digestion and the development of thrush.

Chapter 6

Detox Your Whole Body

We are all exposed to more toxins than we should be – whether by means of pollution or what we actually eat. Regularly detoxifying your body will help you to deal with these toxins.

Tip 26: Take Milk Thistle Before Bed

When it comes to detoxifying the body and supporting liver function, there are few herbal remedies that can match Milk Thistle. Milk thistle is a potent anti-oxidant and speeds toxins from the body.

The high Silymarin content in milk thistle makes it invaluable for preventing liver disease and helping to support an ailing liver. Milk thistle can make some people nauseas so I recommend taking it just before bedtime – it won't keep you awake and can work well while you are sleeping.

With milk thistle, as like most herbal remedies, you should not take it continuously for more than a month at a time without a break. Take if for a month and then have a break of at least two to three weeks before starting up with it again.

Tip 27: Have a Fast Day or Afternoon

Conversely to what you might expect, studies have shown that a lower calorie intake is conducive to a longer life. Having a fast once a week or so allows your body time to recuperate.

There are a few ways that you can go about this. You can either eat nothing all day, eat very bland foods like rice and broth all day or just have a liquid diet.

Choose the method that works best for you. And don't force yourself to do a full day if you find that this is too hard for you. Fasting for the afternoon can also be beneficial if done on a regular basis.

Do choose a day of the week when you are not as busy and do not fast if you are under a lot of pressure. You also need to ensure that you keep well-hydrated during this period. (This not only speeds up the detox but it also helps to keep hunger in check.)

Be prepared, you might feel light-headed or a little ill during this time. This is merely a sign that it is working.

Tip 28: Dry Brushing Your Skin

The lymphatic system in the body has the unenviable task of removing waste from the body. The system is quite efficient but it can become sluggish because it relies on the action of muscles to move the lymph around.

If you are not active enough the lymph system will battle to move the waste that needs to be excreted.

You can stimulate this process by manually moving the lymph. Dry brushing is a good way to do this.

Start with the right brush – you need something that will not scratch the skin but that is firm enough to be able to make a difference. A natural-bristle brush is your best option here.

It is best to do this just before you shower or bath so that old skin cells are washed away immediately.

Starting at your feet, brush firmly in strokes that always move towards the heart. Continue until you reach the shoulders. Do not dry brush your face. Doing this on a daily basis will not take long and will pay dividends in the long-term.

Tip 29: Get into the Bath

Now, I just want to preface this tip by stating that you should not do this if you have high blood pressure or epilepsy.

This bath is very relaxing, it helps to detoxify the body and it can ease sore and tired muscles. The Epsom Salts contain magnesium and this can be absorbed through the skin while bathing.

The baking soda helps to speed up detoxification. Have a hot bath with 2 cups of Epsom salts and half a cup of baking soda in it to help you detoxify and relax the whole body. The water should be as hot as you can manage.

You will need to soak in the bath for at least twenty minutes to get the full effect. Have a glass of water with you in the bathroom and sip whilst bathing.

When you get out of the bath, wrap up warmly and relax – it is best not to schedule anything too demanding after this session. You might even find that you want to go to sleep.

To increase the detoxification effect of the bath, you can also add in essential oils as well. Look into adding the following:

Juniper Berry essential oil will help stimulate the lymph system and speed toxins out of the bloodstream.

All of the citrus oils, like orange, lemon, lime and grapefruit will help to boost immunity and further increase the detoxification effect.

Eucalyptus oil is very helpful in the treatment of muscular aches and pains.

Tip 30: Seek Out Organic Produce and Eat Whole Foods

We are what we eat. The more toxins you put into your body, the more difficult it becomes for your body to deal with them. Lighten the load by choosing foods that are as close to natural as possible.

The fewer additives there are in your food, the easier it will be to for your body to deal with them.

The closer your food is to its natural state, the more nutritious it is bound to be. The more refined the food is, the higher the chance that you are eating empty calories.

Start off by looking for food that has been organically grown. Whilst it may cost a little more, it will be better for your body in the long-run.

If you have the space at home, you could also consider growing your own veggies. Tomatoes, beans, and lettuce will all do well in containers if you don't have the space to make a bed of veggies.

If you cannot grow your own veggies, or you cannot source an organic source, do the next best thing and try to find a local farmer's market to get your veggies from. The vegetables will be more likely to be fresh and the fresher they are, the more appealing they will be.

Others who are considering purchasing this book would love to know what you think. If you could spare a few seconds, they would greatly appreciate reading an honest review from you. Simply visit the page on Amazon.com.

Chapter 7

Create Your Own Spa Treatments

There is nothing quite like spending a couple of days at a spa to help refresh and revitalize you. If your budget won't quite stretch that far, don't worry, there are a lot of spa treatments that you can replicate at home as well.

Tip 31: Start by Recreating the Atmosphere

Spas are designed to be serene places, where you are able to completely relax and unwind. Replicate this in your own home as best you can, whether you are having one spa treatment or a day of pampering.

Start by switching off your mobile phone and unplugging your landline if you have one. Going through the house and switching off all electronic devices like TV's and computers is also a good idea.

Decide where you'll be spending your time and prepare accordingly. Tidy up the bathroom and bedroom so that they are clutter-free and free of distractions. Get everything that you need to get done finished so that you can concentrate on the relaxation.

Do any prep work that you can ahead of time so that you can concentrate on relaxing. Prepare food that you might like to eat and get your drinks ready as well.

If you have kids, get someone to look after them for you while you are having your spa day.

Now get your space ready. Choose some soothing music to play and set up a few candles so that you can switch off all the lights. Scent the bed linen with a relaxing essential oil like Lavender or Sandalwood oil.

You can even pick some fresh herbs to put in the bathwater if you want to. (One tip here, do put the herbs in a muslin bag or a facecloth tied into a pouch. Whilst it might seem awfully romantic to have rose petals in the bath tub, the reality of having to clean them up afterwards detracts from the mood somewhat.)

Tip 32: Create a Salt Scrub to Get All the Dead Skin Gone and Get Circulation Flowing

Exfoliating your skin ahead of time will help to make any treatments that you do apply work a whole lot better. Scrubs can be as simple or as complicated as you like. All you need is a bit of salt or sugar and enough oil to make a paste out of it.

If you like you can also add a drop or two of essential oil. If you are using any oils aside from Lavender or tea tree oil, make sure that you literally only add one or two drops. Essential oils are very concentrated and should not be applied neat to the skin.

Take the time to work the paste into your skin. Again, work from your feet upwards, using firm strokes in the direction of your heart.

The coarser the sugar or salt you use, the more intense the exfoliating action so do keep this in mind when it comes to the sensitive areas of skin like on your face, for example. It is best to stick to a finer-grained sugar for the facial area.

Alternatively, you can use a loofah sponge or dry brushing to exfoliate your skin beforehand.

Tip 33: The Power of the Shower

In Japan, it is customary to climb into the shower and clean yourself before relaxing in the tub. This makes a whole lot of sense and can make your whole experience more pleasant.

Rinse off the scrub properly in the shower before moving into the bath to relax.

Increase the power of the shower by turning it into a treatment in its own right. Alternate bursts of hot and cold water are bracing and improve the circulation in your whole body. It will also help to tighten the pores of the skin.

You can also create your own treatment in the shower itself. Take a clean wash cloth and dampen it. Drop a few drops of the essential oil of your choice onto it and place it on the floor of the shower.

The heat from the shower will help to disperse the scent and it will become a treatment in its own right.

Tip 34: Turning Your Bath into A Spa Treatment

In the chapter on detoxification, I gave you a treatment to use in the bath. As this is a relaxing treatment, you can use it under this section as well.

There is more to hydrotherapy though and you can use this to your advantage. If the idea of soaking in the tub does not appeal to you, you can try a sitz bath instead.

There is a cautionary note when it comes to the sitz bath, it is not a good idea if you have high blood pressure.

You will need two large basins that you can sit in for this treatment. Fill one with cold water and one with water as hot as you can stand. Sit in the cold bath and place your feet in the hot bath. Stay like this for about ten minutes and then switch. This boosts the circulation in the body and helps to build up your immunity as well.

If you do like to soak in the tub, light some candles, put on some of your favorite music and add essential oils or your favorite bubble bath to the tub.

Keep the windows closed and the bathroom door closed and run a hot bath. The steam from the water in the room will add a further treatment element.

If you are adding essential oils, do so only once the bath has been drawn.

Tip 35: Making Your Own Masks

Part of what makes a spa such a special experience is the rich face and body treatments that they offer. You can do something similar at home for a fraction of the cost.

What I do recommend is keeping the treatments to your face and neck only. Full mud treatments for the body are great but they can be particularly messy in your home. The Epsom salt bath will soften the skin very nicely and is nowhere near as messy to clean up.

If you do not want to use the Epsom salts, you can also increase the treatment value of the bath by adding a cup of whole milk to it. If you are using essential oils, mix them in with the milk so that the fat in the milk disperses the oils first.

Face masks can easily be made at home and most times you will have the ingredients you need in your cupboard.

A raw egg is great for toning the skin. A mashed up avocado or a mixture of banana and honey will give you a great moisturizing treatment.

And don't throw away those papaya skins from breakfast either. They make an ideal skin toning treatment. (Do a patch test on the skin before trying this ahead of time.)

Clay treatments are great for controlling oily skin. You can find fine Kaolin clay at the drugstore or at some department stores.

Mix it with enough water to form a smooth paste and apply to the skin. Allow it to dry completely before rinsing it off with tepid water.

Chapter 8

Getting Better Quality Sleep

There is nothing like a good night's sleep to put you on the right track again. These tips will help you get a great night's sleep.

Tip 36: Setting the Stage for Sleep

The first step to a better night's rest is to set the stage for sleep. Start off by clearing out as much clutter from the bedroom as possible. Clutter is extremely distracting. Even if your conscious mind does not register it, your sub-conscious mind will and it will prevent you getting a restful night's sleep.

The next step is to make sure that your bedroom is as dark as possible. Take out any appliances that have a LED light – like your alarm clock or DVD player. Use blackout blinds to cut out as much light as possible.

Next, you need to reduce extraneous noise as far as possible. This is not quite as simple as keeping the room dark, especially if you live in a noisy area. You might want to consider getting a set of earplugs to drown out the noise.

Tip 37: Reducing Your Exposure to Blue Light Before Bed Time

I love surfing the internet and I used to do so until the early hours of the morning. Then I would wonder why I couldn't sleep. Research has shown that exposure to blue light, like the kind of light emitted by the TV, computer or mobile phone, has the same suppressing effect on melatonin production that sunlight has.

Basically, what this means is that it interferes with your ability to fall asleep. The best way to stop this is to switch off all appliances and to dim electric lights at least an hour or two before going to bed.

That is not always an option so an alternative is to wear a pair of sunglasses in the evening to cut out those rays of light. It sounds weird but it really does work – try it.

Tip 38: Go to Bed Earlier

You know how your mother used to nag you to go to bed earlier. It turns out that she was right. Going to bed later and getting up later can land you the same amount of sleep as going to bed early does. Research has shown, however, that the sleep before 12 o'clock at night is more restorative.

Tip 39: Go to Bed When You Are Sleepy

You know how sometimes you are very tired but you stay up anyway and get a second wind? The reason that you get that second wind is because the body releases cortisol to help you stay awake.

This is very damaging to your system because it means that more cortisol is coursing its way around your body. Don't ignore your body's natural sleep cycle.

Tip 40: Stop Worrying About Lack of Sleep

Not being able to fall asleep when you think you should is disconcerting. The problem is that you could end up winding yourself up to a point where you actually can't sleep.

Lying in bed worrying about not getting enough sleep is counter-productive. For starters, we tend to underestimate how much sleep we are actually getting.

Secondly, even if you are not sleeping, the fact that you are lying in bed does help your body to effect some of the repairs that it needs. It is thus not the end of the world if you do not fall asleep quickly.

I hope you have learned something from this book so far and would greatly appreciate it if you could leave an honest review on Amazon.com.

Chapter 9

Lotions and Potions

Tip 41: Increased Vitality Using Essential Oils

Aromatherapy has been used as a healing treatment since ancient times. It can help to boost immunity, fight disease and help your mind heal as well.

You only need two or three bottles of essential oils in your home kit. All essential oils contain some anti-bacterial properties. Choose essential oils that you enjoy the smell of to give you a physical and mental boost. The easiest way to use essential oils is in a diffuser – this will help the scent permeate the house.

Here are some you might like to try:

- **Lavender:** A good all-round oil. Good to use at night to help you sleep, to relax you or to cure a headache.

- **Eucalyptus:** This is the oil to clear congestion fast.

- **Sandalwood:** This has a soothing effect on the mind and can help when you are battling to sleep.

- **Neroli:** A very uplifting oil.

- **Lemon/Lime:** These are great to give you a wake-up jolt in the morning.

Tip 42: Using Natural Skin Care Products

The fewer chemicals you expose your body to, the better for you. You can quite easily make your own skin creams using a mixture of aqueous cream and essential oils or fresh herbs.

Lavender oil/ fresh is very soothing for all skin types. You can also consider using chamomile essential oil as it is one of the few herbs to contain Azulene – a compound that tones the skin.

Other good oils/ herbs to consider are Rose-Scented Geranium, Palmarosa, Sandalwood, and Rose.

To make your own creams, use a concentration of no more than 2% - 3% when it comes to essential oils. It is easier to use essential oils because all you need to do is mix them in. You also don't need to worry about the mixture turning rancid.

When it comes to fresh herbs, use about a cup of the herb to a cup of aqueous cream. Heat the cream and the herb in a double boiler and let it simmer for twenty minutes.

Cool and strain before using. Add two capsules of the oil from a Vitamin E supplement to reduce the chances of the cream going off.

Tip 43: Herbal Tea Recipes

I have spoken about the benefits of herbal teas in a previous chapter.

In this one, I will give you a few recipes that you can try out on your own. These teas can be enjoyed hot or cold, depending on your personal preference.

All the recipes used here use fresh herbs. If you use dried in place of fresh, just halve the quantities. If you are going to drink the tea warm, allow the herbs to seep for at least five to ten minutes. If you will be drinking the tea cold, leave the herbs in the water until it cools before straining.

Afternoon Zinger

For those times that you need an extra boost of energy without the jitters that go with caffeine, try this tea. I find that it is particularly good iced and make a big pitcher of it the day before I need it.

- 3 bags of Rooibos/ Red Bush tea
- 3 bags of green tea
- 1/2 cup of fresh mint
- Honey or sugar to taste
- A pitcher of boiling water

Indigestion Tea

If you have a touch of indigestion, this tea will soon put you to rights. This one is enough for one cup.

- ¼ fresh mint (I like black/ peppermint best for this)
- A few sprigs of Lemon Verbena
- 1 cup of boiling water

Soothing Tea

Again, this is enough for one person. This tea will help you unwind if you are wound up.

- ¼ cup rose petals (An old-fashioned scented rose, not a hybrid)
- ¼ cup of rose-scented geranium flowers
- 1 cup of boiling water

Anti-Flu Tea

- Juice of half a lemon
- 2 teaspoons peeled and finely sliced ginger
- 2 teaspoons of honey
- 1 cup of boiling water

Tip 44: Massage Oils to Keep You Healthy

Massage is extremely healing, especially when combined with aromatherapy. When it comes to aches and pains, nothing works quite as well as a good massage.

Using essential oils as a first aid treatment can help you to recover naturally without the reliance on harsh, synthetic chemicals.

Having said that, if you are in severe pain, or if it does not lessen after you have applied the blends, do go and see your doctor to get it checked out.

The instructions for the following recipes are all the same. Mix together well and apply to the areas that need it.

The following essential oil blends will help to keep you healthy.

Pain-Killing Blend

This is great for when you have a toothache, headache or stiff muscles. If you are using it for a toothache, apply only to the outside of the cheekbone – never use essential oils internally.

- 5 drops Lavender oil
- 5 drops Roman Chamomile oil
- 100ml carrier oil like grapeseed oil or sweet almond oil

Sore Muscle Soother

Don't use this recipe too close to bed-time as the peppermint oil can be quite stimulating. If you need a night-time recipe, switch out the peppermint oil for lavender oil.

- 5 drops Eucalyptus oil
- 5 drops peppermint oil
- 100ml carrier oil like grapeseed oil or sweet almond oil

Circulation Booster

- 5 drops sweet orange oil
- 5 drops juniper berry oil
- 5 drops eucalyptus oil
- 150ml carrier oil like grapeseed oil or sweet almond oil

Night-Soother

- 5 drops lavender oil
- 5 drops roman chamomile oil
- 5 drops ylang-ylang oil
- 150ml carrier oil like grapeseed oil or sweet almond oil

Tip 45: It's All About the Honey, Honey

One magical ingredient when it comes to promoting good health is honey. Now I realize that honey is full of carbs but the benefits of taking it regularly outweigh the potential downside. All you need to promote good health is a teaspoonful a day. If you have that at the same time as you are eating a good meal with a lot of fiber in it, the impact on your blood sugar will be negligible.

Honey is one of the most nutritious foods on the planet. It has natural antibiotic, antiseptic and antiviral properties. In fact, its antibacterial properties are so strong that honey that was found in tombs in Egypt was still edible a few thousand years after it had been put there. Honey will help to build immunity and help to fight viruses and bacteria as well. It feeds the good flora in the gut and can help to restore normal gut function if you are ill.

Honey is great for when you have colds or flu – it can help to fight the infection, provide electrolytes to replace what has been lost and also soothe a sore throat or a cough. It is best to source raw honey where you can and to use that. Honey on the comb is even better for you.

Chapter 10

General Pick-Me-Ups

Tip 46: Add Some Turmeric

If you suffer from chronic pain, a turmeric or curcumin supplement may be just what the doctor ordered. You can try to use more turmeric in your day to day cooking but the truth is that you will not be able to get enough of the active ingredient, curcumin, to do enough good this way.

To maximize your uptake of curcumin, look for a supplement that also contains pepper or eat a couple of peppercorns when you take your supplement. Pepper boosts the amount of curcumin that your body is able to absorb and use.

For pain, turmeric can be considered one of nature's superstars. In scientific trials, it was found to be as effective as NSAIDs. The bonus is that it is all-natural and does not have all the side effects.

Turmeric has been used in Ayurvedic medicine for centuries as both a pain reliever and general health tonic. It is one of the best cures for indigestion – just mix about a teaspoonful in a half glass of milk and it will soothe heartburn quickly.

Do make sure that you take your supplement with food as it is a lot more concentrated than plain turmeric powder.

If you have gallstones, you should not take a turmeric supplement because it can stimulate bile flow and thus cause problems for you.

Tip 47: Cinnamon Please

Is there anything quite like cinnamon on pumpkin pie or fresh pancakes? Cinnamon shouldn't be reserved just for the holidays, though – it is a great health booster all year round as well.

Cinnamon can help to stabilize your blood sugar levels. Just 2g a day can be as effective as anti-diabetes drugs like Glucophage. In fact, this can be so effective that, if you are taking Glucophage, you need to monitor your sugar levels every day or you could end up with low blood sugar instead.

Speak to your doctor about giving cinnamon a try if you are currently on diabetes medication but do not stop taking your medication without consulting your doctor. If you have been diagnosed as pre-diabetic and are at the stage where the disease can be staved off with the right diet, taking cinnamon daily could help you win the fight.

How you take the cinnamon is up to you. You can either wolf it down in one go or sprinkle it over your food – the choice is yours.

Tip 48: Build Your Social Network

Humans as a species were designed to be social creatures. At some point or another, all of us want to feel as though we belong. When it comes to maintaining good health, the importance of having a good social support structure cannot be overemphasized.

You need someone that you can celebrate with, someone that you can talk to – social interactions are a valuable way to alleviate stress. Even though it may seem, at times, that they cause anxiety. How many times have you wanted to avoid a social event, only to find that you actually had a really good time?

It is important to have people that you can lean on in times of crises but also just as important to have people who rely on you. Doing good things for others gives us a boost that we simply can't get any other way.

If you truly want to be content in your life, you need to know both that there are people that you can rely on and that you can also be relied on if the situation calls for it.

Tip 49: Take Good Care of Yourself

This one would seem like good common sense but it is amazing how often we neglect it. Perhaps you are running around helping others or simply too involved in your own life to look after yourself properly.

It is time to begin to be a little more selfish. After all, what good are you going to be if you burn yourself out? What good would you we be if you become ill? How much would you be able to do for others and yourself at such a time?

Taking care of yourself is about more than just diet and exercise, though that is a big part of it. You need to make sure that you have things in your life that you do only for you. You need to make sure that you have at least one activity in your life that you look forward to and you need to learn how to say, "No" to others.

Taking care of yourself allows you to recharge your own batteries so that you can truly be there when there is a real emergency. Take care of yourself – you are just as important to those around you as they are to you – what they want you to do over the long-term?

Tip 50: Ditch the Sugar

I have left this one for last because, of all the tips, I believe that this is the most challenging. Sugar tastes good and it is in just about everything that we eat so it is easier said than done when it comes to quitting.

What you may not have known about sugar is that it is truly addictive – when you have a "fix" it affects the same pleasure centers in your brain that drugs do. As you use more and more, you develop a tolerance for it just as you do for drugs and you crave it more and more.

And sugar is nothing but empty calories and, whilst it may not work as fast as cocaine, it is just as deadly.

When you have a sugary snack, the pleasure centers are activated so you feel good. Unfortunately, the effect on your body as a whole is far from good. Sugar is converted into glucose very quickly by the body and you have a resultant spike in your blood glucose levels.

Your body produces more insulin to cope with the sugar and your body is flooded with insulin and your energy levels plunge. You crave more energy quickly and so you reach for another sugary snack.

Now, if this happened only occasionally, it wouldn't be a problem – the body would get rid of the excess insulin.

The problem is that it happens too often. The body becomes flooded with insulin so often that it becomes less sensitive to the effects of insulin overall. More insulin needs to be produced to have the same effect.

Insulin is a hormone and it causes your body to store the excess glucose as fat in the liver, in place of burning it. It also causes a hormonal imbalance in your body and you get caught in a vicious cycle.

Ditch the sugar now – it simply is not worth having in the long run.

Don't forget to share your thoughts on this book by leaving a review on Amazon.com. It takes just a few seconds.

Are You ALWAYS Hungry When You Try to Lose Weight?

Discover How to STOP Starving Yourself & Lose Weight FASTER By Eating MORE Food!

For this month only, you can get Kayla's best-selling & most popular book absolutely free – *The Ultimate Guide to Healthy Eating & Losing Weight Without Starving Yourself!*

Get Your FREE Copy Here:
TopFitnessAdvice.com/Book

Discover how you can **start eating MORE food** and see weight loss results faster than ever before. Learn about the 10 most powerful fat-burning foods and how they boost the rate that your body burns fat. And last but not least, finally put an end to your emotional or "bored" eating habits. With this book, readers were able to significantly improve their weight loss results. So, it's highly recommended that you get this book, especially while it's free!

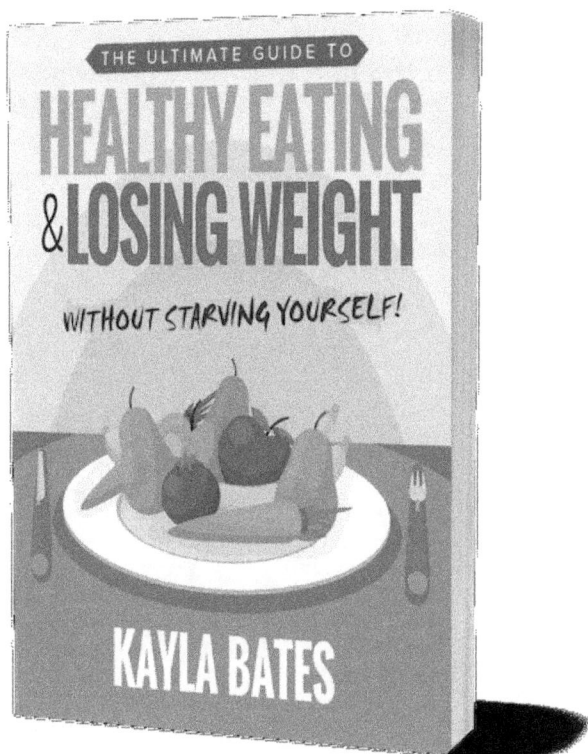

Get Your FREE Copy Here:

TopFitnessAdvice.com/Book

Conclusion

Well, we're done!

I do hope that you found these tips useful and that you have already started implementing the ones that apply to you in your own life.

If you have, I am sure that you have started to see results. As you start to use more and more of the tips, you will see the benefits snowball. With a little bit of effort, you can regain the vitality of your younger days.

Disease and fatigue are not the norm when it comes to the way that our bodies were designed. We tend to accept it as the norm now because we don't know any better. Take back your life and live the way that you were always meant to.

I wish you the best of luck in your own personal journey!

Enjoying this book?

Check out my other best sellers!

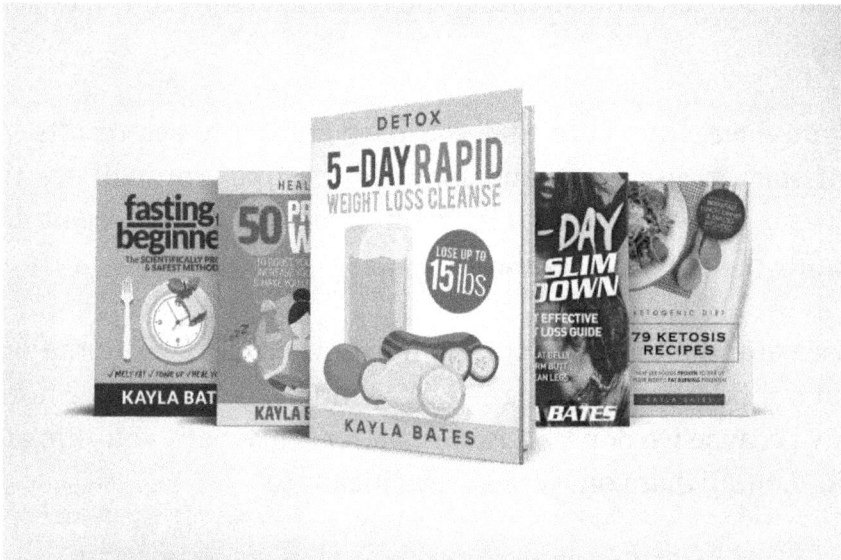

Get your next book on sale here:

TopFitnessAdvice.com/go/Kayla

Final Words

I would like to thank you for purchasing my book and I hope I have been able to help you and educate you on something new.

If you have enjoyed this book and would like to share your positive thoughts, could you please take 30 seconds of your time to go back and give me a review on my Amazon book page.

I greatly appreciate seeing these reviews because it helps me share my hard work.

You can leave me a review on Amazon.com.

Again, thank you and I wish you all the best!

www.ingramcontent.com/pod-product-compliance
Lightning Source LLC
Chambersburg PA
CBHW031206020426
42333CB00013B/806

9 781925 997415